CBD-RICH HEMP OIL

Copyright © 2018 Laura K. Courtney

All Rights Reserved. No part of this book may be reproduced or used in any form or by any means without written permission from the author.

TABLE OF CONTENTS

Introduction 7

Chapter One 10

    What is Cbd Oil? 10

    Is Cbd Marijuana? 12

    How Cbd Works in Our Body 14

    Health Benefits of Cbd 16

Chapter Two 25

    How to Use Cbd Oil 25

    Methods of Extracting Cbd Oil 29

How to Make Your Own Cbd Oil 31

Chapter Three 41

Cannabis Therapies 41

Cannabis Dosing 50

Dosage Guidelines 55

Cbd Side Effects and Drug Interactions 58

Chapter Four 60

Legality of Cannabis 60

What to Look For in Your Cannabis Medicine 63

Cbd Misconceptions 66

Cannabis Oil Vs. Hemp Oil 78

Chapter Five 80

What is Hemp Seed Oil? 80

Hemp Seed Oil Uses 84

Hemp Seed Oil Nutrition 87

Chapter Six 91

Hemp Seed Oil Benefits 91

Hemp Seed Oil Dosage 97

Can Hemp Oil Make You High? 97

Hemp Seed Oil Side Effects 99

Other Books by The Author 104

INTRODUCTION

Thank you for choosing this book, '*CBD-Rich Hemp Oil – The Healing Power of Cannabis medicine: How to Extract, Use and Heal with CBD Oil for Better Health.*'

Cannabis is one of the most versatile plants in nature and yet considered unlawful in most parts of the world. Also known as CBD or marijuana, it has just as many debates surrounding its use. However, it is unfortunate that most of the controversies surrounding cannabis and its uses are clouded with confusing and incorrect information.

CBD oil has been used in medicine for millennia, but the concern over the risks of abuse led to the ban of the medicinal use of cannabis in the 1930s. Marijuana and related compounds are being considered therapeutic only recently. An outstanding compound, cannabinoid found in cannabis or CBD is responsible for the medicinal and psychoactive effects of the plant and has shown to be capable of curing several ailments.

In this guide, you'll learn all you need to know about the powerful medicinal effects of CBD-rich hemp oil;

including its numerous health benefits where just a little goes a long way in improving general wellness. You will also find simplified information to help you understand exactly how you can use CBD-rich hemp oil to improve your health.

CHAPTER ONE

What is CBD Oil?

The CBD oil acts as a natural remedy and perfect alternative for soothing many health problems. CBD is also referred to as cannabidiol, which is a compound found in the cannabis plant. The oil works together with the endocannabinoid system found in the human body. The endocannabinoid system performs a significant role in the most of the rational body functions. The CBD oil contains two important compounds – CBD and little amounts of THC so it doesn't lead to the "high" feelings.

Is CBD Marijuana?

CBD oil, which is also known as cannabinoid, is one of the compounds obtained from the cannabis plant. Until recently, the most popular compound found in cannabis was delta-9 tetrahydrocannabinol (THC), which is the most active ingredient in marijuana.

Marijuana has both CBD and THC however, the compounds possess different effects. THC is popularly known for the mind-altering (high) effects it gives when it is broken down by heat and ingested into the body like when cooking it into food or smoking the plant.

However, CBD is not psychoactive like THC. In other words, CBD doesn't change the state of mind when used and it has been found to have significant health benefits. The CBD that is used medicinally is obtained from the least processed form of the cannabis plant, called hemp.

Marijuana and hemp are derived from the same plant, known as cannabis sativa, but they're very different. Over the years, farmers of marijuana have carefully grown their plant to be high in THC and other compounds they prefer, either for the effect they had on the plant's flowers or the aroma. On the other hand, farmers of hemp have not tried to alter the plant. And these hemp plants are used to produce CBD oil

How CBD Works In Our Body

All cannabinoids as well as CBD, link themselves to particular receptors in our body to generate their effects. The body creates cannabinoids naturally and it possesses 2 receptors for cannabinoids, referred to as CB1 and CB2 receptors.

CB1 receptors are present in all parts of the human body, but most of these receptors are found in the human brain. The receptors found in the human brain work with memories, appetite, thinking, mood and emotions, pain, and movement and coordination, among others. THC connects to these receptors.

CB2 receptors are commonly found in the immune system. They affect pain and inflammation. Until recently, it was believed that CBD acts on the CB2 receptors, but it has been revealed that CBD doesn't act on either receptor directly. Rather, it appears to help the body to use more of its own cannabinoids.

Health Benefits of CBD

CBD is a medicinal herb and is well-known for its numerous benefits, which includes:

1. **Anti-inflammatory and natural pain relief properties**

People typically make use of over-the-counter or prescription medication to alleviate stiffness and pain, which includes chronic pain. Nonetheless, many people have found CBD to offer a more natural way of reducing pain. According to a study published in the Journal of Experimental Medicine, CBD drastically lower chronic pain and inflammation in some rats and mice during experiment. The researchers proposed that the non-psychoactive compounds found in marijuana, like CBD, could be used to treat chronic pain.

2. Epilepsy and other mental health disorders

CBD has been studied for its potential characteristic in treating epilepsy and neuropsychiatric disorders. According to a review posted to Epilepsia, CBD is said to have anti-seizure properties and a low risk of adverse effects for people who suffer from epilepsy. More studies on the effects of CBD on neurological disorder have shown that CBD may help to treat most of the disorders, such as psychiatric diseases, neuronal injury, and neurodegeneration that are associated with epilepsy. In another study, published in Current Pharmaceutical Design, it was found that CBD may have the same effects as certain antipsychotic drugs and that it may be effective and safe to be used for treating patients with schizophrenia. However, more research is required to really understand how this works.

3. Quitting smoking and drug withdrawals

There's some promising proof that shows that CBD may help people to give up smoking. A pilot study published in Addictive Behaviors established that smokers who used inhalers containing CBD compounds smoked fewer cigarettes and didn't experience any additional yearning for nicotine. A similar study published in Neurotherapeutics has found that CBD may be a great substance for people who abuse opioids. Some researchers have found that some symptoms felt by patients who suffer from substance use disorders may be reduced by CBD. Such symptoms include insomnia, pain, mood symptoms, and anxiety. They also suggested that CBD might be used to reduce or avoid withdrawal symptoms.

4. Fights cancer

CBD has been found to have anti-cancer properties. According to a review published in the British Journal of Clinical Pharmacology, CBD seems to help prevent cancer cells from spreading around the body and invading a new area. This review shows that

CBD tends to repress the growth of cancer cells and aid the death of these cells. Researchers also found that CBD may be used in cancer treatment due to its low toxicity levels. Therefore, they requested for it to be studied along with standard treatments, to test for synergistic effects.

5. Type 1 diabetes

The type 1 diabetes occurs as a result of inflammation that happens when the immune system attacks the cells that are found in the pancreas. A recent study published in Clinical Hemorheology and Microcirculation shows that CBD may help to relieve the inflammation in the pancreas in type 1 diabetes. This could be the first step in finding a CBD-based treatment for type 1 diabetes.

6. Anxiety disorders

Patients who suffer from chronic anxiety are usually advised to stay away from cannabis since it can cause or increase anxiety and paranoia in some people. Nevertheless, a review from Neurotherapeutics proposed that CBD may help to ease the anxiety experienced by people who suffer from certain anxiety disorders. The researchers referred to the studies that indicate that the compound may help to relieve anxiety behaviors in disorders such as:

- obsessive-compulsive disorder

- social anxiety disorder

- panic disorder

- general anxiety disorder

- post-traumatic stress disorder

The review found that the current medicines for the above disorders can result in additional side effects and symptoms and that the patients may have to stop taking the medications due to the unwanted side effects. CBD hasn't shown any side effect in any of those cases to date, and the researchers have requested for CBD to be studied as a possible treatment method.

7. Alzheimer's disease

An early research posted to the Journal of Alzheimer's Disease established that CBD was able to prevent the development of social recognition deficits in patients. In other words, CBD may possibly prevent patients in the early stages of Alzheimer's from losing their ability to recognize the people they know. Therefore, this is the initial proof that the compound has the ability to avert Alzhcimer's disease symptoms.

8. Acne

The usc of CBD for acne treatment is very promising. Acne is partly caused by overworked sebaceous glands and irritation in the body. A new research published in the Journal of Clinical Investigation shows that Cannabis helps to reduce the generation of sebum that causes acne, partially due to the anti-inflammatory effect it has on the body. It is believed that CBD may be a potential remedy for acne vulgaris, the most common form of acne.

CHAPTER TWO

How to Use CBD Oil

CBD oil can be used in many ways to alleviate the symptoms of various conditions. Some CBD oil products can be used as a thick paste to be massaged into the skin, taken from a dropper or pipette, or mixed into foods or drinks. CBD is also available in capsule form. There are other products produced as sprays that can be administered under the tongue.

Below are some recommended dosages, though the dosage may differ among people based on other factors, like the condition being treated, the concentration of the product, and body weight. Make sure you seek medical advice before deciding on any particular dosage due to lack of FDA regulation for CBD products. All dosages should be taken by mouth:

- **Glaucoma**: One dose of between 20 mg and 40 mg CBD administered under the tongue can ease pressure in the eye. Although, caution is strongly advised since dosages greater than 40 mg may increase pressure.

- **Schizophrenia**: Take between 40 mg and 1,280 mg CBD per day by mouth for about four weeks.

- **Sleep disorders**: Consume between 40 mg and 160 mg CBD per day by mouth.

- **Movement problems associated with Huntington's disease**: Consuming 10 mg daily for 6 weeks can help to reduce movements.

- **Epilepsy**: Take between 200 mg and 300 mg CBD per day by mouth for about 4.5 months.

- **Chronic pain**: Consume between 2.5 and 20 mg of CBD by mouth for no more than 25 days.

More prescriptions and precise doses will start to surface as the laws surrounding CBD in the U.S. increases. After discussing with your doctor about the dosage and risk involved, as well as researching regional legal use, it is essential that you compare different brands. There is a variety of different CBD oils to buy online, with different applications and benefits.

Methods of Extracting CBD Oil

There are three main methods of extracting the CBD oil which include:

- **CO2 Method**: This process involves pushing the CO_2 through the cannabis plant at a high pressure and low temperature. Through this method, the purest form of CBD oil is extracted. It's the safest and most refined method of neatly extracting the CBD oil, removing compounds like chlorophyll and ensuing in no residue. The oil obtained from the CO_2 method has a cleaner taste; however, it is an expensive technique.

- **Oil Method**: This technique is the most popular and it involves the use of carrier oil for extraction of CBD. The olive oil is commonly used for this method. It is becoming quite popular because of the additional benefits of nutrients from carriers oils. The oil method is also safe and will not produce any residue.

- **Ethanol method**: This technique of extracting CBD oil involves the use of high-grain alcohol. However, the ethanol method destroys a little amount of beneficial natural oils.

How to Make Your Own CBD Oil

CBD is gaining recognition all over the world due to its medicinal properties. There're various ongoing studies and research about the use of CBD oil. CBD or cannabidiol is an ideal cure for alleviating the symptoms of many medical conditions. The cannabis plant is used to extract the CBD oil. This oil has many benefits which include providing relief for chronic pain, MS, schizophrenia, epilepsy, PTSD, alcoholism, arthritis, and diabetes. The CBD oil is anti-inflammatory, anti-spasmodic, anti-nausea, and analgesic treatment that works great for most people.

Many individuals are searching for answers concerning the connection of CBD oil and medical conditions. In history, cannabis had been in use for the treatment of illnesses until it was made unlawful. The cannabis plant has two most significant compounds – CBD and THC. THC causes the "high" or "drunk" feeling while CBD helps to relief most of the symptoms because of its medicinal properties.

Oil method

This CBD oil recipe works effectively for dermatitis, arthritis, psoriasis, lupus, and others due to its decongestant, analgesic, and anti-inflammatory properties.

Ingredients

- 14 grams of organic leaves and buds of CBD

- 1 cup of carrier oil e.g. 50% extra virgin olive oil, 25% coconut oil, or 25% almond oil

Instructions

- First of all, blend the buds, leaves, and stems of the cannabis plant in a coffee grinder.

- Then, decarboxylate the ground leaves and buds by baking for 90-100 minutes at 220°F

- Place the oil in a glass jar, add the ground cannabis plant to it and cover tightly.

- Place a dish cloth in a saucepan and place the jar on the it.

- Add about 2 to 3 inches of water in the saucepan

- Boil the water at 200°F for approximately 3 hours. Once the water starts to reduce, add more to the saucepan to prevent it from drying up.

- Carefully shake the glass jar few times after an hour but be cautious because the jar would be very hot at that point.

- After 3 hours, turn off the heat and place a towel on the sauce. Allow cooling for 3 hours.

- Then repeat the above process. You may repeat the process for the next three days to produce stronger oil but you can make use of the product after one day.

- Strain the oil from the herbs with cheesecloth into another jar or container. Make sure you squeeze the cheesecloth well to obtain the most from the cannabis plant.

- You can use the finished product for local purposes, to discover the changes you will experience in your body.

Alcohol method

CDB or other cannabinoids can be effortlessly extracted using alcohol which is an easy and safe process. When using this system of extraction, you don't need to make use of any special skill or equipment for the production of powerful CBD oil. This method is also considered to be the best for the extraction of CBD oil since it doesn't leave any harmful or unpleasant residue.

Ingredients

- 4 liters of alcohol

- 30 grams of ground Cannabis buds

Equipment

- Ceramic or glass bowl

- Funnel or plastic syringe and wooden spoon or silicon spatula

- Catchment container

- Double boiler

- A fine strainer for example; nylon stockings, cheesecloth, or sieve

Instructions

- Start by preparing the equipment and cleaning the working area.

- Place the cannabis buds in a bowl and cover with the alcohol. Stir the mixture for about three to six minutes with a wooden spoon to expel the resin.

- Ensure the container you are using can hold the solvent and raw material.

- Use a sieve to filter the solvent and take out the raw extraction into a container. Squeeze out as much liquid as possible.

- You may repeat the process of filtering and squeezing with a new batch of alcohol solvent to extract adequate CBD oil.

- Place your extracted liquid in a double boiler. Heat up the liquid until it begins to bubble. Let the alcohol evaporate without increasing the temperature.

- Turn the flame to low heat and let the mixture simmer for 15 to 30 minutes lightly. Continue to stir and don't let the liquid to get heated up.

- Once the alcohol has evaporated completely, combine the extracted fluid and scrap it with a silicon spatula.

- Place the concentrated CBD oil in a storage bottle or select a dosage container before the CBD oil turns thick and cold with time.

- Pull the oil in a plastic syringe and store in a dark, small sealed container. You may also segment the dose by using toothpicks or a small spoon or by squeezing a small quantity of CBD oil from the plastic syringe.

CBD oil extracted with the use of grain alcohol is a safe and effective technique, which is highly suitable for consumption.

CHAPTER THREE

Cannabis Therapies

Cannabis remedies are available in various forms and can be used in many ways. The most suitable delivery system for curative cannabis is the one that offers the best dosage for a preferred duration with fewer side effects.

1. **Cannabis Oil Extracts**

Cannabis oil extracts can be consumed sublingually, orally, or applied topically. The potent CBD oil extracts can also be used to cook or vaporize. A few CBD oils come with an applicator for measured dose. The oil extracts such as THC-dominant and CBD-rich are very effective. The period of commencement and length of effect differ depending on the mode of administration.

2. Smoked cannabis

Cannabis is usually smoked in a joint or pipe. When cannabis is breathed in, THC, CBD, and other compounds get absorbed by the lungs, into the blood, and across the blood-brain barrier. The initial outcome of inhaled cannabis typically happens within a few minutes of inhaling it and slowly wears off after two to three hours. Smoking cannabis is usually effective for the treatment of acute symptoms, such as nausea, vomiting, and painful spasms, which require urgent treatment. It's relatively easy to titrate the dosage by inhaling. If the result is inadequate after a few minutes, another puff can be taken until the desired effect is attained. However, smoke has noxious compounds that might irritate the lungs.

3. Vaporizing

Vaporizing cannabis with devices such as vape pen provides the same immediate effects as smoking. However, a vaporizer heats the cannabis oil or flower without burning it; only the active ingredients are inhaled as a vapor without smoke. Therefore, this process is a healthier alternative to smoking.

4. Edibles

Cannabis edibles are foods that are cooked with cannabis-infused oil, ghee or butter. The effects of cannabis taken orally can linger for about 4 to 6 hours, which is significantly longer than inhaling cannabis. However, the beginning of the effects is much slower (30-90 minutes) compared to sublingual sprays or inhaled cannabis. Therefore, the slow onset and longer duration make this therapy more suitable for the treatment of chronic health problems that need a stable dose of medication all through the day. The major hazard of taking cannabis orally is the issue of overconsumption. And the longer duration makes it hard to titrate the dosage. Therefore, it is advisable for one to proceed carefully by consuming a small dose of an edible and waiting at least one hour before determining if more is needed or not. Consuming edibles might be suitable for an individual suffering from lack of appetite, vomiting or nausea.

5. Juices

Raw cannabis juice produces with a food processor or blender will have THCA, CBDA, and other non-psychoactive cannabinoids because it is also not heated. It's hard to determine an exact dosage using this method, yet the health benefits are potentially important.

6. Tinctures

The tincture is an herbal remedy that makes use of the active ingredients of cannabis dissolved in alcohol or another solvent. The result, effect, duration, and dosage are similar to those of edibles.

7. Sublingual Sprays

These sprays are produced from cannabis extracts which have been mixed with an additional substance such as coconut oil. This concentrate is sprayed beneath the tongue and rapidly absorbed through the oral mucosa. The initial effects of this therapy are typically felt within five to fifteen minutes of using it. A Sublingual spray is a great alternative for discreet, consistent, and timely cannabis dosing. It doesn't involve any preparation or lingering smell from smoking.

8. Cannabis Teas

When cannabis is prepared as an herbal tea, it will contain considerable amounts of THC and CBD in its raw "acid" form (THCA and CBDA) since the heat needed to steep tea is less than the temperature required for "decarboxylation," which changes THCA into THC and CBDA into CBD. Cannabis tea is not intoxicating due to the fact that cannabinoid acids do not connect with receptors in the brain. THCA and

CBDA seem to contain considerable therapeutic properties; however, there has been little research on the compound.

9. Capsules & Gel Caps

Cannabis oil can also be administered in a capsule or gel cap such as supplements and vitamins. The dosing, duration, and effect are similar to those of edibles.

10. Cannabis Oil Extracts

Cannabis oil extracts can be consumed sublingually, orally, or applied topically. The potent CBD oil extracts can also be used to cook or vaporize with. A few CBD oils come with an applicator for measured doses. The oil extracts such as THC-dominant and CBD-rich are very effective. The period of commencement and length of effect differ depending on the way of administration.

11. Topical & Salves

Cannabis oil and tinctures can be infused in an ointment, lotion, or balm and rubbed directly on the skin. Many people have reported that cannabis topical is very effective for skin conditions, infections, inflammation, and pain. Since they're applied externally, salves and topical are not intoxicating.

Cannabis Dosing

Personalized Medicine

Cannabis therapeutics is a personalized medicine. The correct treatment routine depends on the patient and condition that is being treated. Select cannabis products that have both THC (tetrahydrocannabinol), the psychoactive component of cannabis, and CBD (cannabidiol), a non-intoxicating compound for utmost therapeutic benefits. THC and CBD work together to increase each other's therapeutic impacts. They certainly work best together. An individual's sensitivity to THC is a major factor in determining the dose and ratio of CBD-rich medication. Many people benefit from cannabis and can ingest moderate amounts of any cannabis product without getting dysphoric or too high. While some people find THC distasteful. CBD can neutralize or reduce the intoxicating effects of THC. Therefore, a greater ratio of CBD-to-THC means less of a "high" feeling. Finding your ratio is the first step to a successful treatment.

Find your ratio

Dosed cannabis medicine is currently available in the form of edibles, capsules, infused sublingual sprays, concentrated oil extracts, and other products, even though it's banned by federal law. Strong cannabis oil extracts have various ratios of THC and CBD that are standardized to meet the needs and sensitivities of each person.

For pediatric seizure disorders, spasms, depression, and anxiety, most patients at first, find they do well with a reasonable dosage of a CBD-dominant therapy (a CBD:THC ratio of more than 10:1). However, a low THC therapy, though not intoxicating, is not unavoidably the best remedial alternative. A blend of THC and CBD will possibly have a superior therapeutic impact for a broad range of health conditions than THC or CBD alone.

For neurological disease, cancer, and many other diseases, patients may derive benefits from a balanced ratio of THC and CBD. Broad clinical research has found that a 1:1 THC:CBD ratio is effectual for neuropathic pain. Maximizing one's therapeutic use of cannabis may involve a careful, step-by-step process, where an individual begins with small amounts of non-intoxicating CBD-rich medicine, monitors the results, and steadily increases the dosage of THC.

In essence, the objective is to self-administer steady, assessable dosages of a CBD-rich therapy that contains as much THC as an individual is comfortable with.

The Biphasic Effect

Cannabis compounds contain biphasic qualities, which imply that high and low dosages of the same substance can create opposite effects. Large doses of cannabis tend to sedate; small doses stimulate. Too much THC, though not toxic, can increase mood and anxiety disorders. CBD does not have any known adverse side effects at any dose; however, drug interactions can lead to problems. Too much of CBD can be less effective medically than a reasonable dosage. "Less is more" is often the case with regards to cannabis therapy and dosage is very important.

Dosage Guidelines

- **Determine how you would like to take cannabis.** Cannabis oil is available in edibles, capsules, sprays, and other products.

- **Discuss with your doctor.** Proceed cautiously, particularly if you have a history of mental illness, alcohol or drug abuse, or are breastfeeding or pregnant.

- **Be wary of possible side effects.** Cannabis is a safe and forgiving medication. However, it can increase mood and anxiety disorders depending on individual tolerance and delivery method. Other possible side effects are faintness, dizziness and dry mouth.

- **Find your ratio**. Cannabis products come with different amounts of THC and CBD. A high THC and high CBD products are not necessarily better than a strain with a balanced ratio. Discover the right blend to maximize your therapeutic uses of cannabis.

- **Start with a low dosage** particularly if you have little or no experience with cannabis.

- **Consume a few small dosages** throughout the day instead of one big dosage.

- **Make use of the same dose and ratio for several days**. Monitor the effects and if needed regulate the amount and ratio.

- **Don't overdo it.** "Less is more" is generally the case with respect to cannabis.

CBD side effects and drug interactions

CBD is a very safe substance to use; however, people who are taking other drugs need to consult a medical professional about drug interactions, which are more probable when taking high dosages of single-molecule CBD products. When taken adequately, CBD will neutralize cytochrome P450 enzymes temporarily, thus changing how we metabolize a wide range of compounds which includes THC. Also know that CBD is a stronger inhibitor of cytochrome P450 than grapefruit compound known as Bergapten, therefore talk to your healthcare provider to know if grapefruit will interact with your medicines. If grapefruit does, then CBD will most likely do too. Cytochrome P450 enzymes metabolize more than sixty percent of Big Pharma meds. Additionally, people who are on CBD-rich treatment routine should monitor changes in blood levels of prescription medicines, and adjust dosage if needed.

CHAPTER FOUR

Legality of Cannabis

Cannabis is lawful for either recreational or medicinal use in some but not all states. Other states endorse CBD oil as a hemp product without allowing the general use of medicinal marijuana. Laws concerning CBD and marijuana may vary between federal and state level, and the present legislation on

CBD and marijuana in the US can be confusing, even in the states where CBD and marijuana are legal.

There is an ever-changing number of states that do not take marijuana to be legal but have regulations that are directly linked to CBD oil. The laws differ, yet CBD oil has generally been approved as lawful for the treatment of epileptic conditions at different concentrations. Furthermore, different states need different levels of prescription to obtain and use CBD oil. For instance, in Missouri, an individual must prove that three other treatment alternatives have failed in treating epilepsy.

Therefore, before you possess and use CBD oil as a treatment, speak to your local healthcare provider.

They'll be aware of local regulations surrounding usage and safe CBD sources. Also, endeavor to research the laws for your own state, but in many cases, a prescription will be needed.

What to Look For In Your Cannabis Medicine

When you're choosing a cannabis medicine, look for:

- **Cannabis, not industrial hemp**: When you compare hemp to the complete plant cannabis, it naturally has low cannabinoid content. An enormous quantity of hemp plant is needed to produce a little quantity of CBD, increasing the threat of contaminants since hemp, which is a bio-accumulator, pulls contaminants from the earth. The energetic terpenes profile of the complete plant cannabis increases the healing benefits of THC and CBD.

- **Safe extraction**: Steer clear of cannabis products that are pressed with noxious solvents such as hexane, propane, BHO, or other hydrocarbons. Solvent filtrates are particularly hazardous for immune-compromised patients. So, make sure you go for cannabis products that involve a safer technique of extraction such as CO_2.

- **Quality ingredients**: Choose products that have quality ingredients. No artificial additives, trans fats, GMOs, and corn syrup.

- **Lab testing**: Select products that are tested for consistency, and established as free of solvent residues, pesticides, bacteria, mold, and other contaminants.

- **Clear labels:** Look for products that have labels that show the ratio and quantity of THC and CBD per dose, batch number for quality control and manufacturing date.

- **CBD-rich products**: For optimal therapeutic effects, select products that have both THC, the main psychoactive component of cannabis, and CBD, a non-intoxicating compound. THC and CBD work perfectly together, promoting each other's healing benefits.

CBD Misconceptions

With the rising awareness of CBD as a potential remedy, there has also been the propagation of misconceptions. The past year has witnessed a surge of interest in CBD, which is non-intoxicating compound found in cannabis with considerable therapeutic properties. Several internet retailers and commercial start-ups have jumped on the CBD bandwagon, hyping CBD obtained from industrial hemp as the next big thing, miracle oil that can relieve chronic pain, quell seizures, and shrink tumors, without making an individual feel "stoned." However, along with an increasing awareness of CBD as a great remedy, there has been a rise of misconceptions about cannabidiol.

1. **"CBD is medicinal. THC is recreational."**

CBD has received various investigation throughout the world and most often, people say they are looking for "CBD, the medicinal part" of the cannabis plant, "not THC, the recreational part" that gets one high. Truly, THC, "which is the high causer" possesses remarkable therapeutic properties. According to some scientists at the Scripps Research Center in San Diego, THC has been found to inhibit an enzyme intertwined in the creation of beta-amyloid pestilence, the hallmark of Alzheimer's-related dementia. The federal government identifies Marinol (single-molecule THC) as appetite booster and anti-nausea compound, considering it a Schedule III drug, a category kept for medicinal compounds with little potential for abuse. However, the entire marijuana plant, which is the only natural source of THC, continues to be considered as a hazardous Schedule I drug without medical value

2. **"CBD is most effective without THC."** CBD and THC are the power duo of cannabis compounds since they work excellently together. Some scientific studies have found that THC and CBD interact synergistically to increase each other's healing effects. Some

scientists that work at the California Pacific Medical Center, San Francisco found that the mixture of THC and CBD contains a more effective anti-tumoral impact than either of the compounds as a single molecule when tested on breast cancer and brain cancer cell lines. British researchers have established that CBD enhances THC's anti-inflammatory qualities in an animal model of colitis. An extensive research also showed that THC combined with CBD is more effective for neuropathic pain than either compound alone.

3. **"CBD is the good cannabinoid, THC is bad cannabinoid."** The drug warrior's tactical retreat – demonize THC while

continuing to give ground on CBD. Intransigent marijuana prohibitionists are taking advantage of the CBD's good news to further degrade high-THC cannabis, framing tetrahydrocannabinol as the bad cannabinoid, while CBD is taken as the good cannabinoid. Why? This is due to the fact that CBD does not make one high like THC does.

4. **"Psychoactivity is intrinsically an adverse side effect."** A politically right drug war catechism believes that the marijuana high has an unwanted side effect. The Big Pharma is dedicated to creating therapeutically active marijuana-like molecules that won't have the "high" effects – however, it isn't clear why mild

euphoric feelings are inherently negative for a sick or even a healthy person. In ancient Greece, the word euphoria (having health) meant a state of healthiness. The euphoric or ecstatic properties of cannabis, apart from being an objectionable side effect, are extremely connected in the therapeutic value of the plant. Dr. Tod Mikuriya suggested that cannabis should be considered as a medicine that contains some psychoactive qualities, just like most medicines, rather than being taken as an intoxicant that contains few therapeutic qualities on the side.

5. **"Single-molecule pharmaceuticals are better than whole plant medicinal."** The

FG has established that specific compounds of marijuana plant (CBD, THC) possess medicinal value; however, the marijuana plant itself doesn't have any therapeutic worth. The single-molecule blinders by Uncle Sam replicate a political and cultural bias that favors Big Pharm's products. Single-molecule medication is the major corporate method, the FDA-approved method; however, it is not the only method, and it is automatically the best way to gain from cannabis remedies. Cannabis has several hundreds of compounds that include numerous aromatic terpenes, flavonoids, and many trivial cannabinoids as well as CBD and THC. Each of the compounds contains particular therapeutic characteristics, yet when they are combined they produce what is called a holistic "entourage effect," so the healing effects of the entire plant is better than the total of its single-molecule parts. However, the FDA is not in the business of approving plants medicine.

6. **"CBD is CBD – It doesn't matter where it comes from."** It actually matters. The leaves and flower-tops of some industrial hemp strains may be a possible source of CBD; however, hemp is by no means the best source of cannabidiol. Naturally, industrial hemp has less cannabidiol than cannabis. Extracting a little quantity of CBD from industrial hemp

requires enormous quantities of industrial hemp, thus increasing the threat of toxic contaminants due to the fact that hemp is a "bio-accumulator" that pulls heavy metals from the soil. Single-molecule CBD extracted and refined from industrial hemp or synthesized in a lab lacks secondary cannabinoids or vital medicinal terpenes found in cannabis strains. These compounds work together with THC and CBD to improve their therapeutic benefits.

7. **"CBD is legal in all 50 states."** Suppliers of imported, CBD-rich hemp oil assert that it is lawful to sell their products anywhere in the U.S. so far the oil does not contain up to 0.3%

THC. In reality, it is not that easy. Federal law forbids United States cultivators of hemp from growing it for commercial purpose; however, selling of low-THC, industrial hemp products (imported) is allowed in the U.S. if the products are obtained from stalk or seed of the hemp plant, and not from flowers and leaves. The truth is that Cannabidiol cannot be extracted or pressed from hemp seed. CBD can be pressed from leaves, flower, and only a very small amount from the stalk of the hemp plant. When they say CBD is derived from hemp stalk or hemp seed, then credibility may be lacking in the hemp oil start-ups. Very soon, Congress may vote to remove CBD and industrial hemp from the definition of marijuana under Controlled Substances Act. However, such legislation won't be required if CBD obtained from foreign-grown hemp is made lawful all over the U.S.

8. **"The 'CBD-only' laws sufficiently serve the patient population."** About 15 United States state legislatures have approved "CBD-only" or "low THC" laws, while other states are ready to do the same. Some states indicate the diseases for which CBD can be used and limit the sources of CBD-rich products: others do not. Apparently, these regulations permit the usage of CBD-infused oil obtained from cannabis or hemp that measures less than

0.3% THC. However, a CBD-rich therapy with small THC does not work for everybody. Parents of children with epilepsy have revealed that the addition of THC or THCA helps to control seizure in many cases. THC-dominant strains are more potent than CBD-rich products for some epileptic patients. Therefore, the vast majority of patients are not well served by CBD-only laws. They do not need to access just the low THC remedy but a wide range of the entire cannabis plant therapy. With respect to cannabis therapeutics, one size does not fit all and neither does one strain or one product or one compound.

Cannabis Oil vs. Hemp Oil

CBD-rich products, made with organic, whole plant cannabis, are highly recommended since they provide better medicinal benefits and the best safety profile.

CBD products made from industrial hemp typically have many problems which include:

- Refined CBD powder and hemp-derived CBD lack secondary cannabinoids and critical medicinal terpenes in cannabis oil. The compounds interact with THC and CBD to improve their therapeutic benefits.

- Industrial hemp naturally contains less

cannabidiol than CBD-rich cannabis strains; therefore a vast amount of industrial hemp is needed to extract a little quantity of CBD. This increases the danger of contaminants since hemp is a "bio-accumulator"- which means it typically draws toxins from the soil.

- It is against federal law to make use of hemp flowers and leaves for medicinal products. Some entrepreneurs of hemp oil try to bypass this legal obstacle by dubiously claiming that their products were extracted from hemp stalk before importation to the U.S., a grey area of activity at best.

CHAPTER FIVE

What is Hemp Seed Oil?

Hemp oil is extracted from the hemp plant. All the plants found in the Cannabis genus can generate oil, but only industrial hemp is used to make hemp oil most often. This industrial hemp is a variety of hemp that has been refined particularly for industrial production; it contains the smallest amount of the psychoactive substances linked with the genus, most especially THC. Hemp oil is naturally almost free of THC, and it doesn't contain any psychoactive property.

The seeds are believed to produce the best hemp oil, even though the whole plant can be processed for oil. Cold pressed oil that has not been cultivated has a green tint and a rich, nutty aroma. After the hemp oil has been refined, it becomes colorless, and the flavor becomes reduced. There're a variety of packaging formats and a number of uses for it.

One typical use of the hemp oil is in soaps. The oil is also used as a body care product and in lubricants and paints. Many people also utilize hemp oil as a dietary supplement, to take advantage of the high concentrations of its essential fatty acids found in unrefined hemp oil as well as using the oil as a garnish or dressing to enhance nutrition.

Unrefined or natural hemp oil doesn't have a long shelf life. It can go rancid rapidly, except it's stored in a dark container in a refrigerator. Those who use unrefined oil usually buy it in little quantities to prevent it from going bad. This oil is not appropriate for cooking since it has a very low smoking point. The refined version has a long shelf life, but many of its benefits are lost after refining.

Hemp is a controversial crop in some parts of the world because of the concerns about the psychoactive plants in the Cannabis genus. Cultivation of hemp is banned in some states, but the products obtained from hemp like oil, hemp paper, and hemp garments may be legal. In other states, only industrial hemp is allowed, and some countries freely allow the cultivation of all the plant in the Cannabis genus, assuming that regulation is a more effective approach for control than complete bans. In addition, wild hemp is common in most parts of the world, making it hard to implement bans on hemp crops.

Hemp Seed Oil Uses

Every application that makes use of petroleum for its hair and skin products can utilize hemp oil since it's more therapeutic and herbal. Hemp oil can also be used for many health problems as a pain reliever or even as its cure.

- Since hemp oil is natural, it can be used as moisturizing oil that can be applied to a bath or a shower. When it is massaged into the body, it helps to nourish the skin and improves blood circulation.

- Another way hemp oil can be used is as biodiesel similar to other vegetable oils. It is really a safe replacement for petroleum since it's non-toxic and harmless to the environment.

- Hemp oil can be used in cooking, although it's not appropriate for high heat cooking. It does not only add a slightly crispy and nutty taste to food but also serve as the perfect salad oil if you run out of olive oil.

- Paints can be produced from hemp oil since it does not lead to any toxic releases when it is washed down the drain and produced very low emissions compared to petroleum paints.

- Hemp oil can be used to make almost all kinds of plastic instead of making use of petroleum as a base. The plastics produced from petroleum do release dangerous chemicals during decomposition but those made from hemp oil don't.

Hemp Seed Oil Nutrition

The oil that can be found in the hemp seed is seventy five to eighty percent of polyunsaturated fatty acids, which are known to be good fats and only nine to eleven percent of the less preferred saturated fatty acids. This oil is presumed to be the most unsaturated oil obtained from the plant kingdom. Additionally, the essential fatty acids found in the hemp oil are needed in daily diet more than any other vitamin, but the human body does not produce them naturally. They must be gotten from external sources in our diet. Essential fatty acids are responsible for producing life's energy in the human body and life is not possible without them. Generally, North Americans suffer from nutritional deficiency in essential fatty acids as a result of the high consumption of animal fats against plant fats as well as the high intake of processed meats and foods versus natural foods.

A broad research has found that many common diseases are associated with imbalances or deficiencies of certain fatty acids in the human body. Symptoms are usually linked to a lack of Omega 6 and Omega 3 fatty acids and their derivatives, which are the prostaglandins. Most individuals that consume a healthy diet, which includes a balanced ratio of essential fatty acids, have a strong immune system and healthy skin. However, some people do experience deficiencies in certain fatty acids or their metabolites as a result of dysfunctional enzyme systems or other inhibitions that occur in their metabolic paths induced by environmental factors or immune-system-related. It has been established in various clinical studies that nutritional supplementation with essential fatty acids or their metabolites usually cures or prevent these diseases. Hemp seed oil has both essential fatty acids in a perfect balance and it also provides two of the essential fatty acid metabolites, which makes it a great resource for the treatment and prevention of certain diseases.

Hemp oil has been termed "Nature's most perfectly balanced oil," because it has the completely balanced 1:3 ratio of Omega 3 essential fatty acid to Omega 6 essential fatty acids, meant to be the optimal necessity for long-term healthful human nutrition. Additionally, hemp oil contains smaller quantities of three other polyunsaturated fatty acids in stearidonic acid, oleic acid, and gamma-linolenic acid (GLA). The EFA blend is unique among edible oil seeds.

Hemp seed oil offers a sufficient supply of phospholipids, carotene (precursor to Vitamin A), antioxidants (Vitamin E), and a number of minerals which include phosphorus, potassium, sulfur, magnesium, calcium, along with moderate amount of zinc and iron. Hemp oil is also a good source of chlorophyll.

CHAPTER SIX

Hemp Seed Oil Benefits

The hemp seed oil has numerous health benefits. Its raw forms and products help to give the body loads of essential amino acids. If the body gets deprived of any the essential amino acids, then there may be serious problems like cancer and genetic mutations. Hemp oil helps to cure cancer since the essential and non-essential amino acids are in abundance in the oil, therefore, when this oil is frequently used for cancer patients, there're possibilities of healing. Hence, hemp seed oil is indeed beneficial for many reasons.

1. Hemp oil benefits for hair

Hemp oil has many health benefits for the hair. Most herbal and non-commercial hair products such as shampoos, conditioners, hair oils, etc. are produced from hemp oil. Massages with hemp oil products can aid blood circulation in the head and brain. Washing the hair with hemp oil conditioners and shampoos can keep dandruff away from the scalp, thicken the hair texture, and improve hair growth. Therefore, hemp oil has great benefits for the hair. It also helps to reduce and prevent hair loss and scalp infections and other related problems.

2. Hemp Oil Benefits for Skin

The hemp seed oil has numerous fatty acids that are great for the skin. The fatty acids help to moisturize and nourish the skin in an adequate amount and the right manner. There are many skin products such as body creams and face creams that use hemp oil as the main ingredients. This is due to the fact that it's herbal and has almost no side effects. Using hemp oil for a skin massage will leave you with a healthy and nourished skin which feels and looks young. Hemp oil also has anti-aging benefits and prevents skin disorders like dry skin, acne, eczema, and psoriasis.

3. "Super" Polyunsaturated Fatty Acids

This amazing oil is loaded with "super" polyunsaturated fatty acids, most especially stearidonic acid and gamma-linolenic acid. These aren't essential fatty acids, yet they can relieve the signs of atopic dermatitis and other skin problems. Nonetheless, the quantity of the non-essential fatty acids differs according to the amount of the hemp plant the fatty acids are gotten from.

4. Alpha-Linolenic Acid

Hemp oil is a great source of alpha-linolenic acid, which is an omega-3 fatty acid that is vital for good organ function. According to the University of Maryland Medical Center, Alpha-linolenic acid is similar to the omega-3 fatty acids found in fish oil and it can be used to relieve depression, arthritis, and heart disease. It also helps to decrease low-density lipoprotein cholesterol, which is the "bad" cholesterol that obstructs arteries.

5. Protein Content

According to Dr. Andrew Weil, the program director for the Arizona Center for Integrative Medicine, hemp seed oil contains 25% protein and this is documented by the Arizona Board of Regents. This oil has high-quality protein which provides amino acids in ratios that are similar to the protein contained in eggs and meats. The composition of the hemp oil proteins makes them effortlessly edible.

When compared to other oils, the hemp seed oil gives the amino acids and protein needed by the body without adding needless calories

Hemp Seed Oil Dosage

The recommended daily dosage of hemp oil is 14-28 ml, about 1-2 tablespoons. The dosage gives you between 3 to 6 grams of Omega 3 (LNA) and between 8 to 16 grams of Omega 6 (LA).

Can Hemp Oil Make You High?

Hemp seed oil does not give the "high feeling". For you to grow marijuana, you must have the special seed that grows into THC high plant, the quality responsible for the drug reaction. Hemp oil has very little amounts and it has a substance that neutralizes THC.

In a nutshell, hemp seed oil is a considerably popular product, which is used for an increasing variety of purposes. However, washed hemp seed does not have THC at all. The little quantities of THC found in industrial hemp are located in the glands of the hemp plant. Occasionally, during the manufacturing process, some CBD- and THC- containing resin attaches to the seed, ensuing in traces of THC found in the oil produced. The concentration of cannabinoids in the hemp oil is infinitesimal. Therefore, no one can get high from using hemp oil.

Hemp seed Oil Side Effects

Hemp seed oil is as great as a dietary supplement to promote general wellbeing and for treating minor health ailments. Hemp seed oil is known to be one of the most beneficial natural supplements for the body because of its content of essential fatty acids which are beneficial to humans. Nonetheless, you need to know the possible side effects of the hemp seed oil. In that light, make sure you discuss with a medical professional for more information on the side effects of hemp oil

1. THC Effects

A study has found that the hemp oil is obtained from a plant that has a high content of the neurological chemical THC. This chemical can lead to high anxiety, euphoria or hallucinations in the users of the supplement when consumed regularly. Therefore, the hemp oil supplements can have the same effects in some of the patients that use the oil for treating any disorders. It has been suggested that the patents who take the supplement shouldn't consume hemp oil products before driving or operating machinery because of the threat of their hallucinogenic qualities. This is particularly true to people who are extremely sensitive to THC. This can be verified by consulting a medical professional for additional information

2. Digestive Symptoms

Hemp seed oil can cause minor side effects in the digestive system. For instance, a study found that hemp and hemp oil can soften the stools, which usually results in abdominal cramping or diarrhea. Most times, extreme diarrhea can result in malabsorption or increased weight loss. Although more research is required to validate these side effects claims, it's advisable for people with a history of irregular bowel movements or digestive disorders to not consume hemp oil supplements.

3. Peroxides

Do not use hemp oil for frying. Hemp oil must be used in warm and cold food items that can't be heated to 121°F because high heat breaks down polyunsaturated fats in hemp oil into dangerous peroxides. You may use hemp oil as a flavor-enhancer in most recipes but not as an alternative to frying oils. Make sure you keep the bottles of hemp oil firmly closed after using and store in the refrigerator.

4. Effects of the Blood

Another common side effect of hemp oil involves the bloodstream and cardiac system. A study established that hemp oil product can have a direct effect on the anticoagulant qualities of platelets in the blood, usually restraining their production. Therefore, people who are presently getting treatment for cardiac medical issues as well as blood clotting deficiency are strongly advised to avoid hemp oil supplements of any form because of potential symptom complications.

OTHER BOOKS BY THE AUTHOR

1. All Natural Soap Making: Ultimate Guide to Creating Nourishing Natural Soap At Home

For You And Your Family Plus 25 Amazing Soap Recipes

2. Bath Bombs: How to Make Beautiful and Nourishing Bath Bombs At Home Using Cheap and Non-toxic Ingredients, Without Fuss

3. Clean Your Home with 66 Homemade Cleaning Products: A Beginner's Guide to Decluttering And Organizing with Natural Home Cleaning Recipes For A Clean And Organized Home

4. Epsom Salt, Apple Cider Vinegar and Honey Natural Remedies: The Miraculous Benefits and Uses for Healing, Health, Relaxation, Beauty and Home

5. Hair Care and Hair Growth Secrets: A Guide to Longer, Healthier and Beautiful Hair – Including 50+ Natural Hair Care Recipes for Growth, Shine and Repair

6. Natural Healing with Essential Oils: The Complete Reference Guide to Using Essential Oils for Aromatherapy, Beauty, Healing, Health and Home Benefits

Printed in Great Britain
by Amazon